# Health

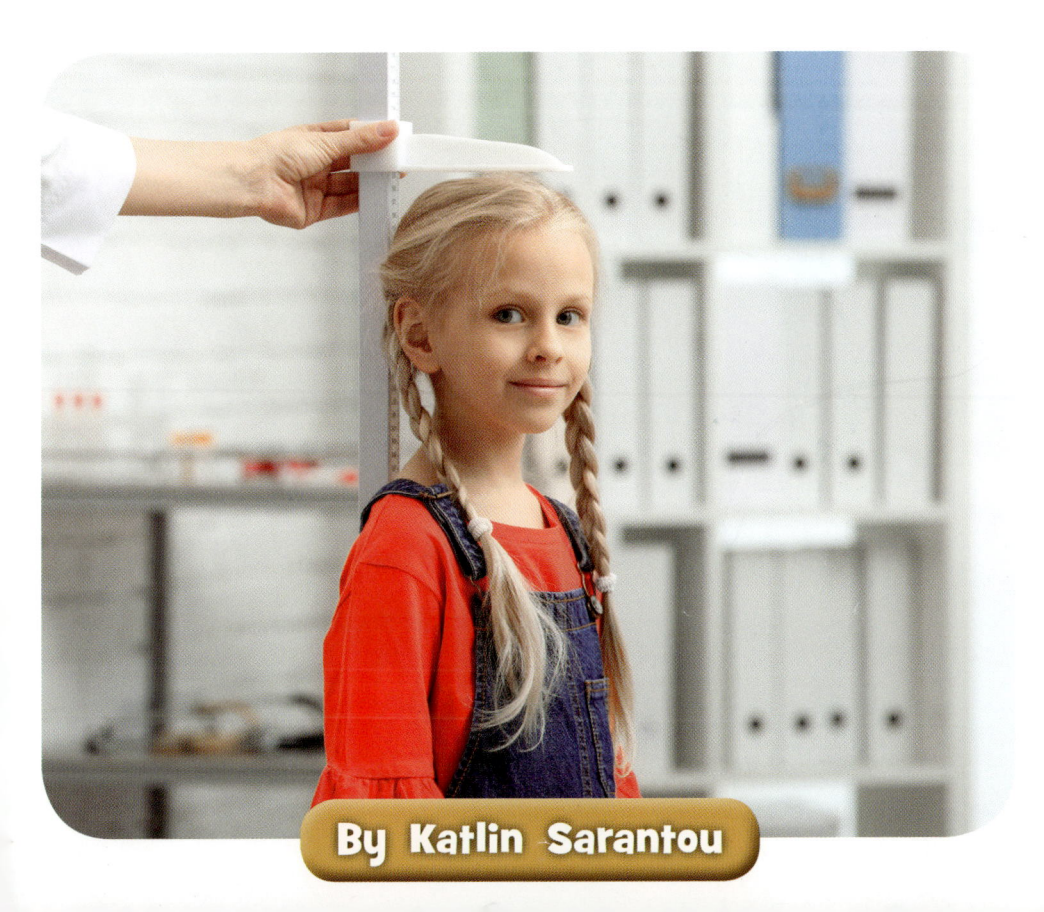

## Visiting the Doctor

By Katlin Sarantou

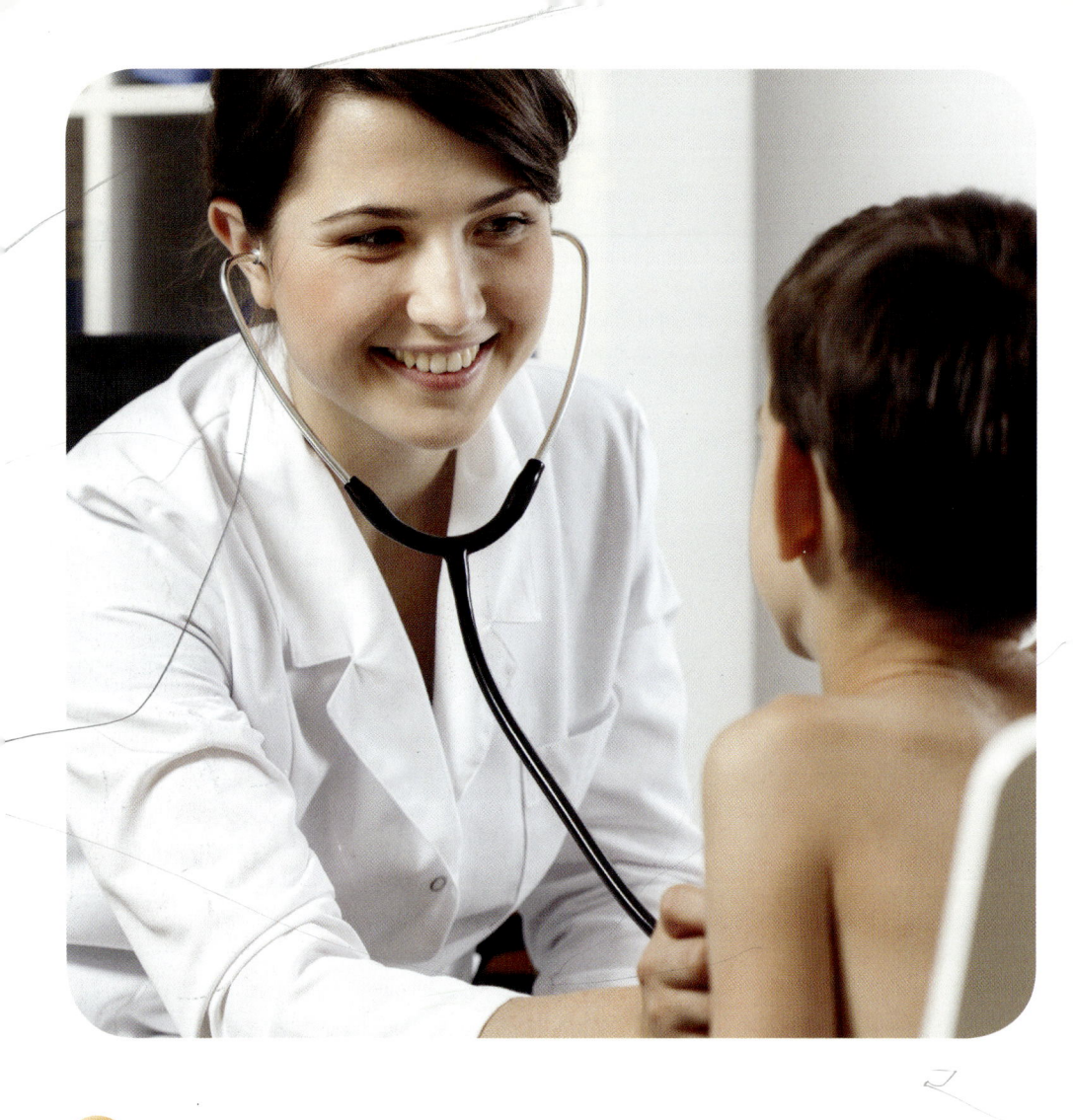

2 The doctor smiles.

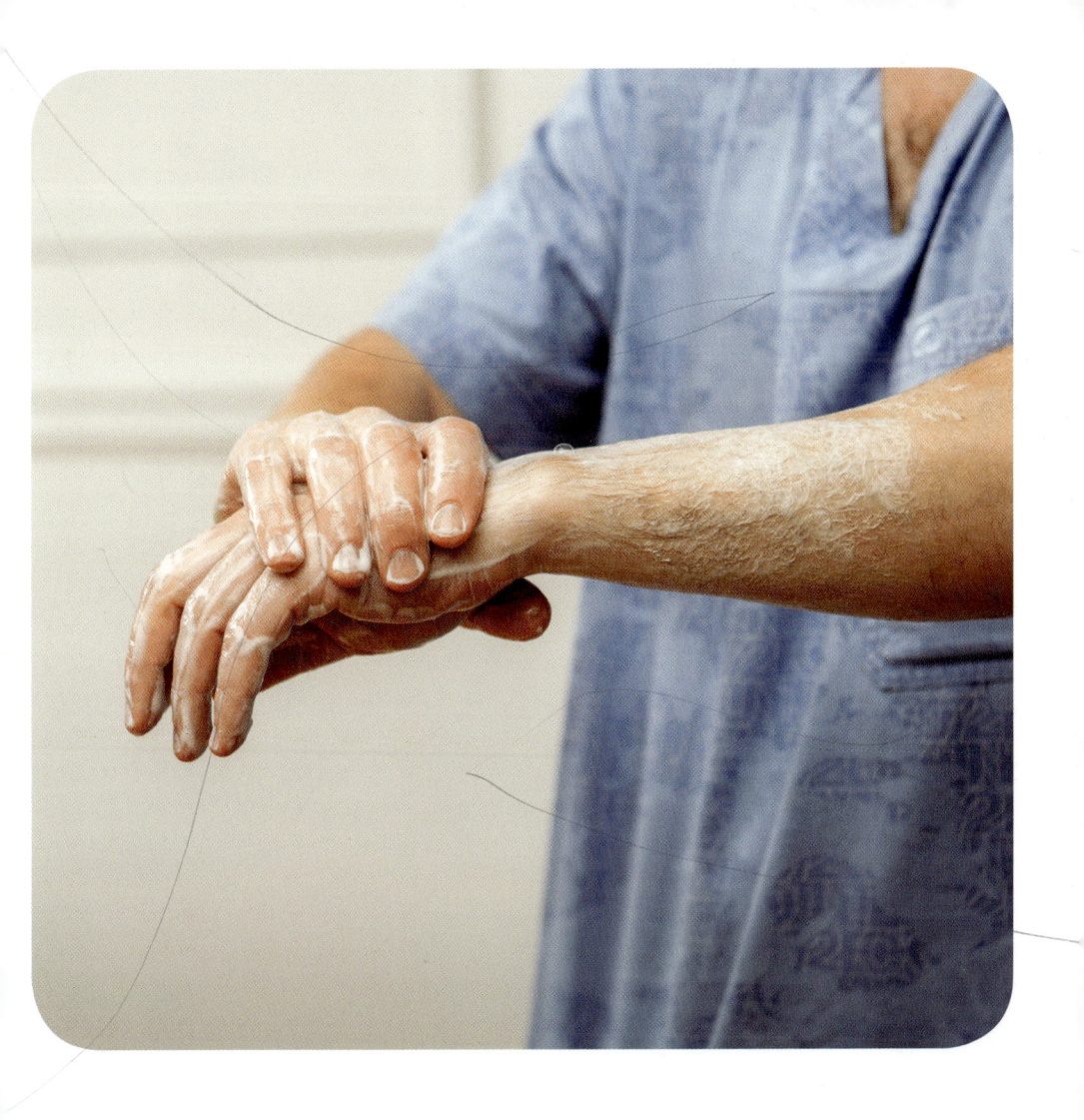

**The doctor washes.**

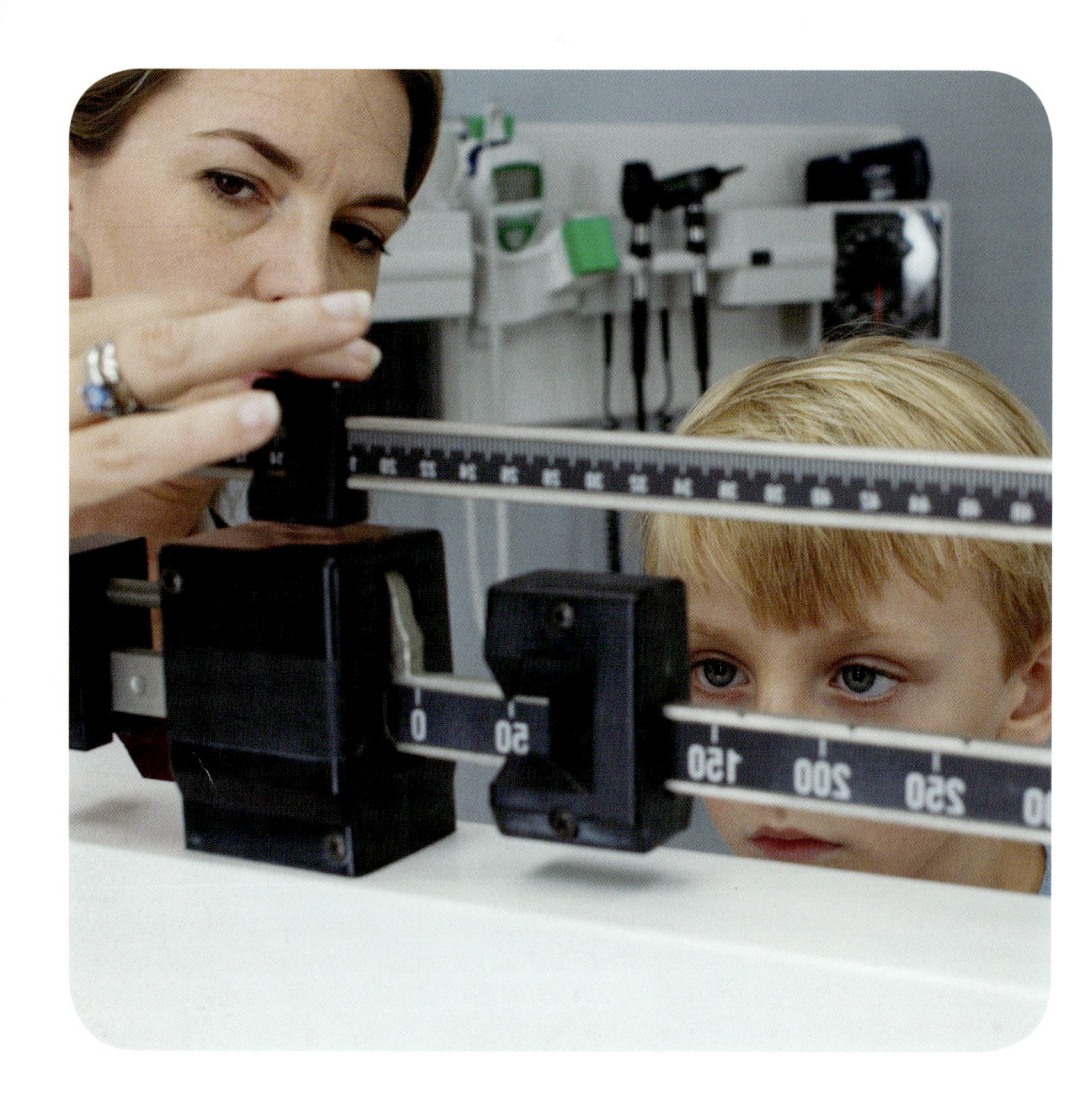

The doctor weighs.

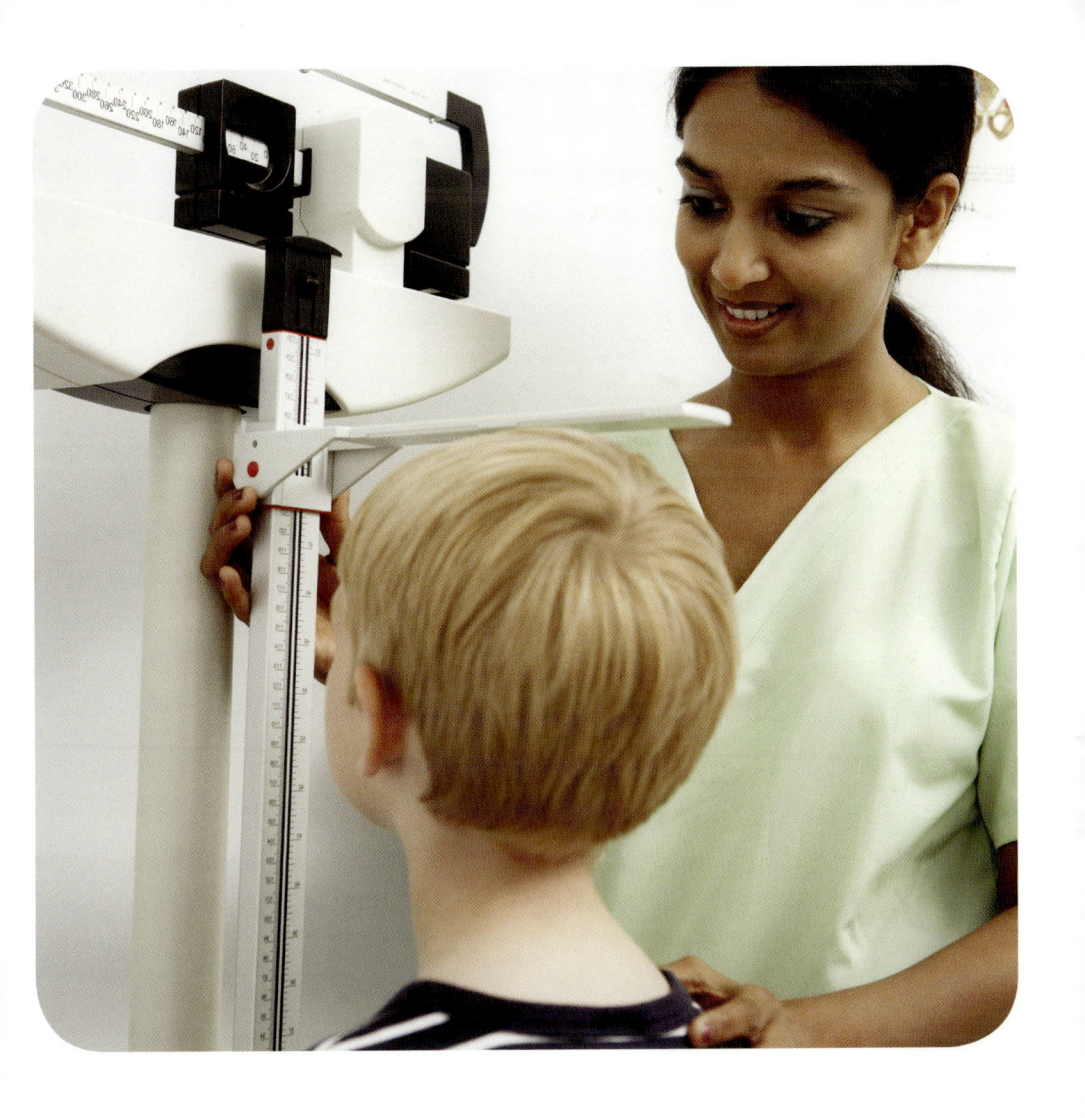

**The doctor measures.**

5

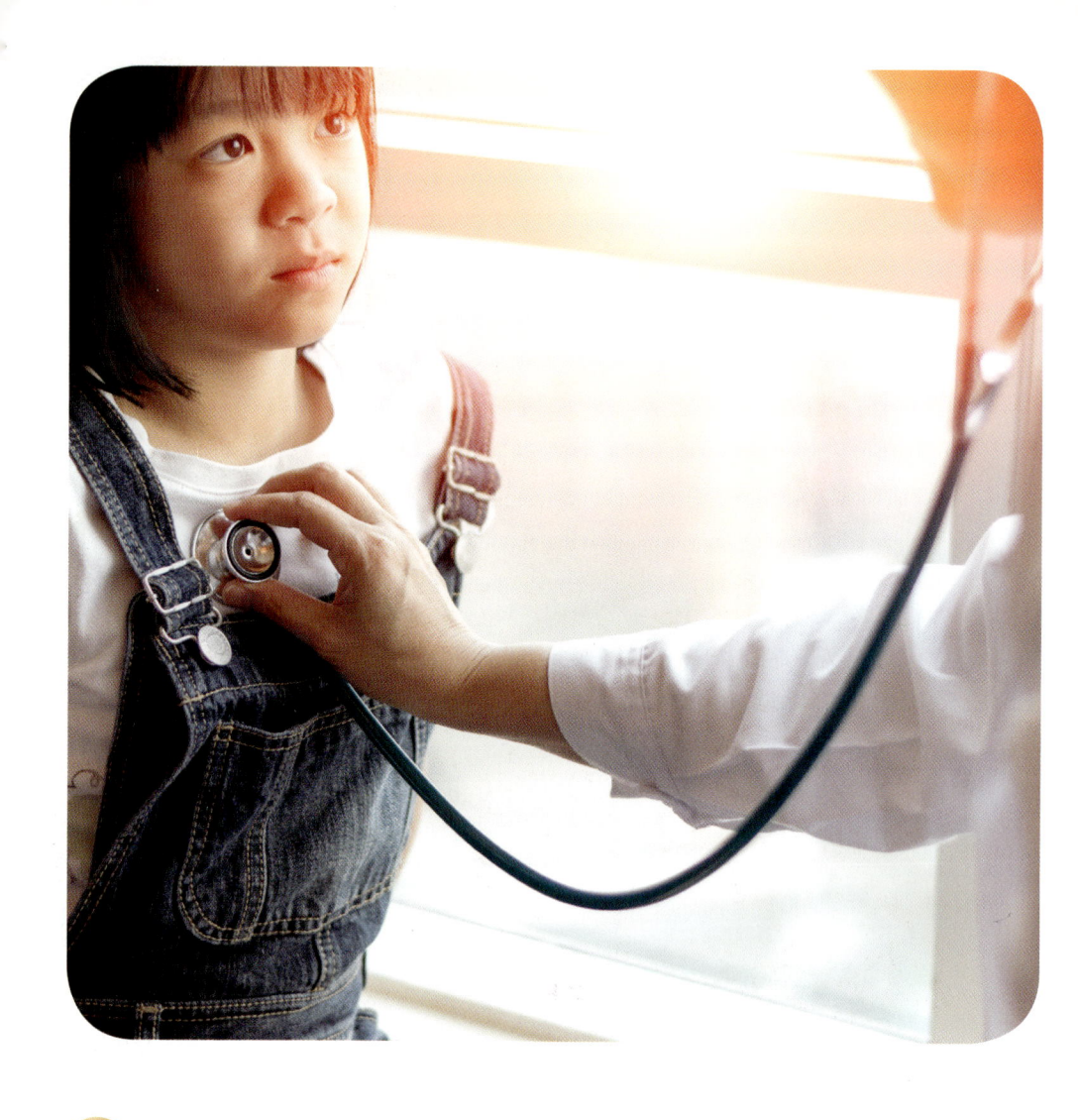

The doctor listens.

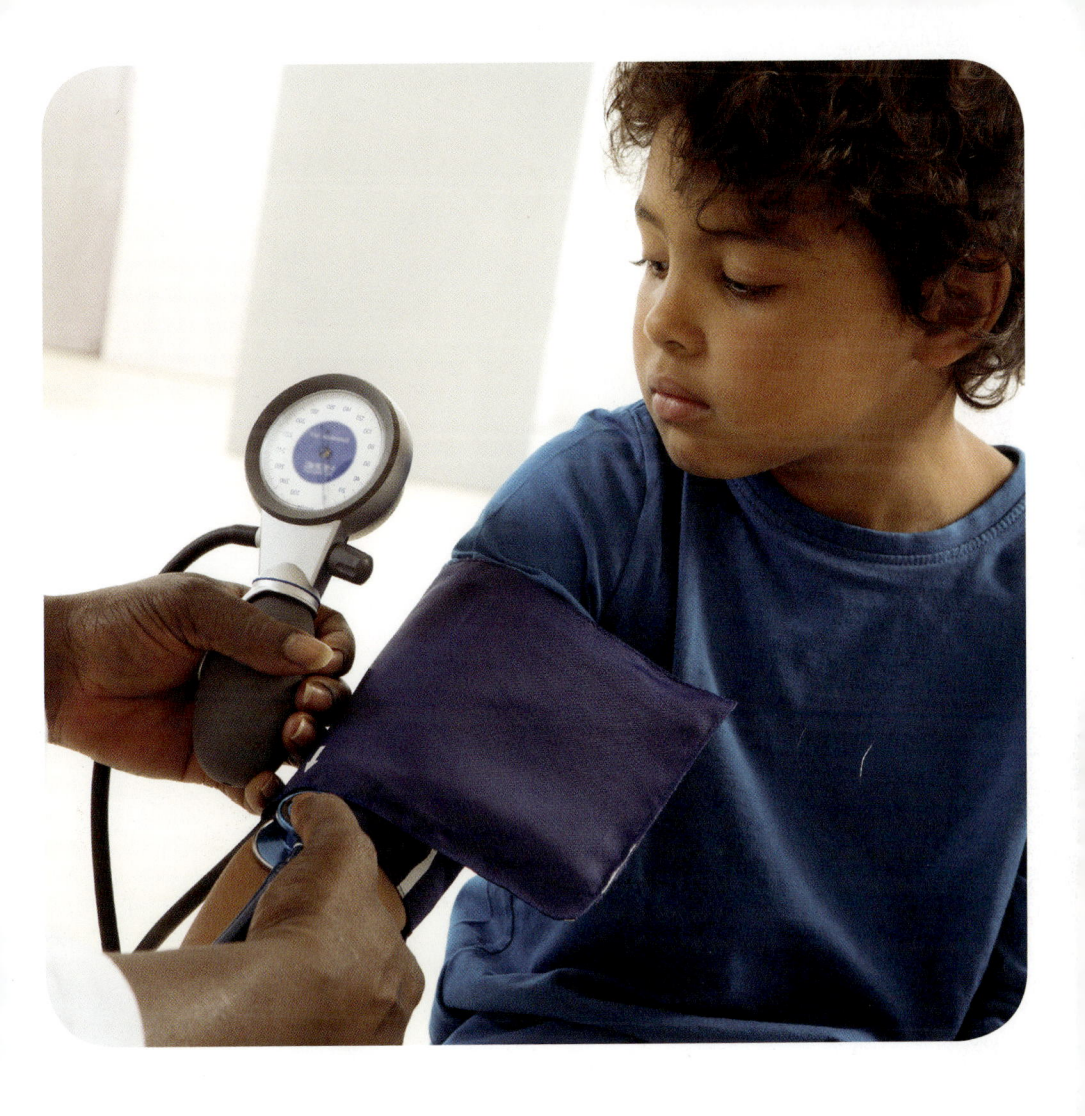

The doctor squeezes.

7

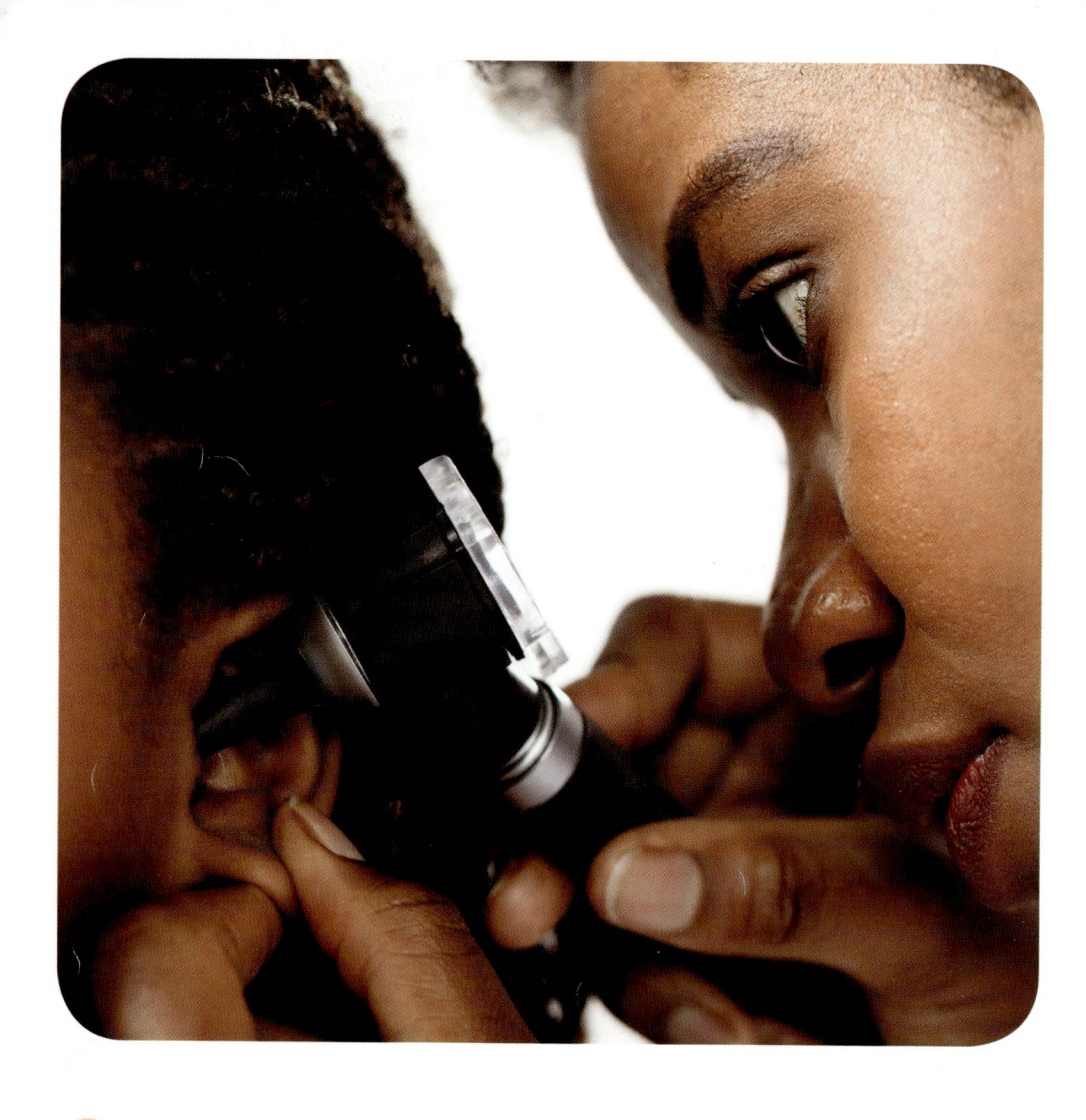

The doctor looks.

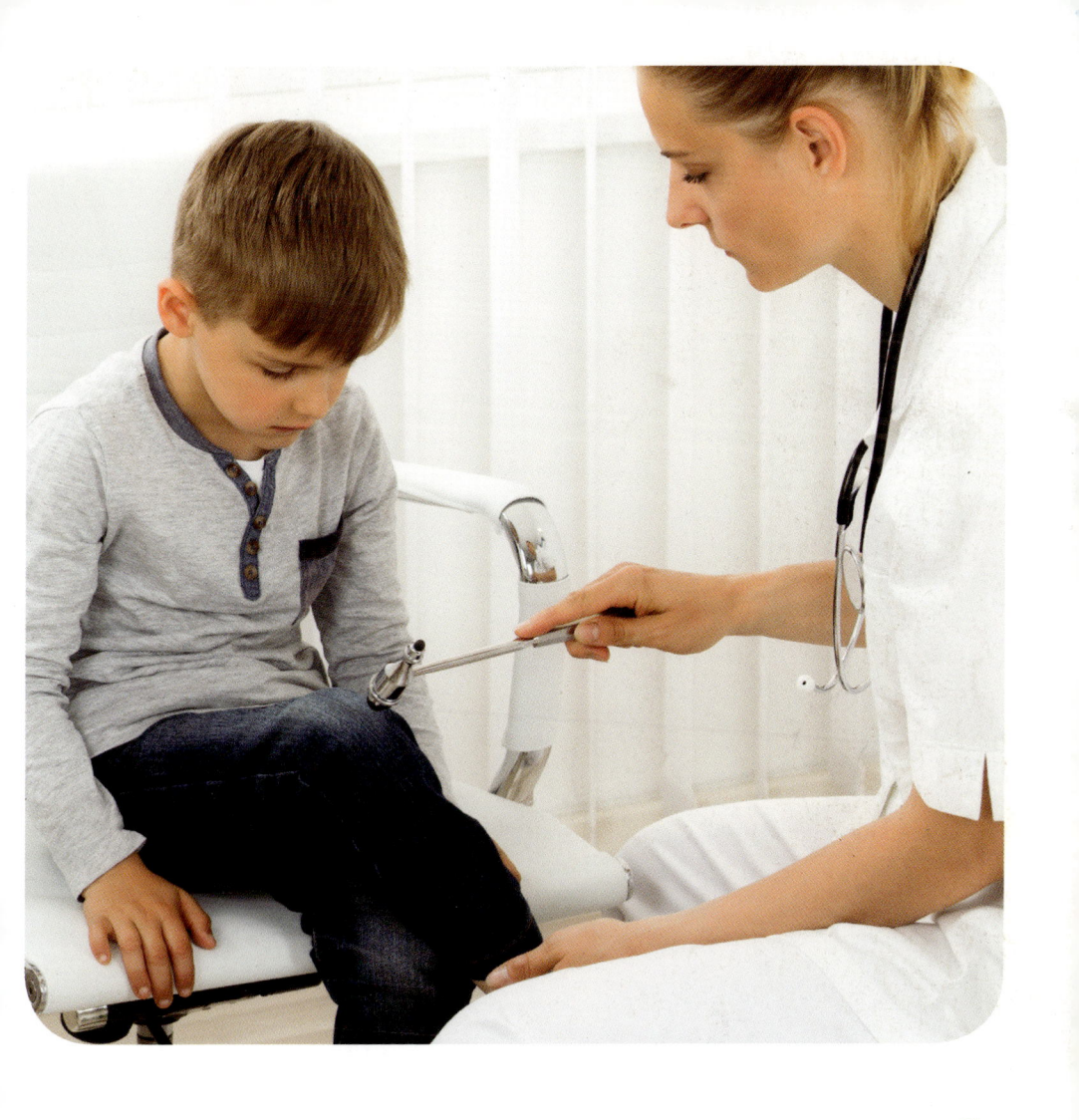

The doctor taps.

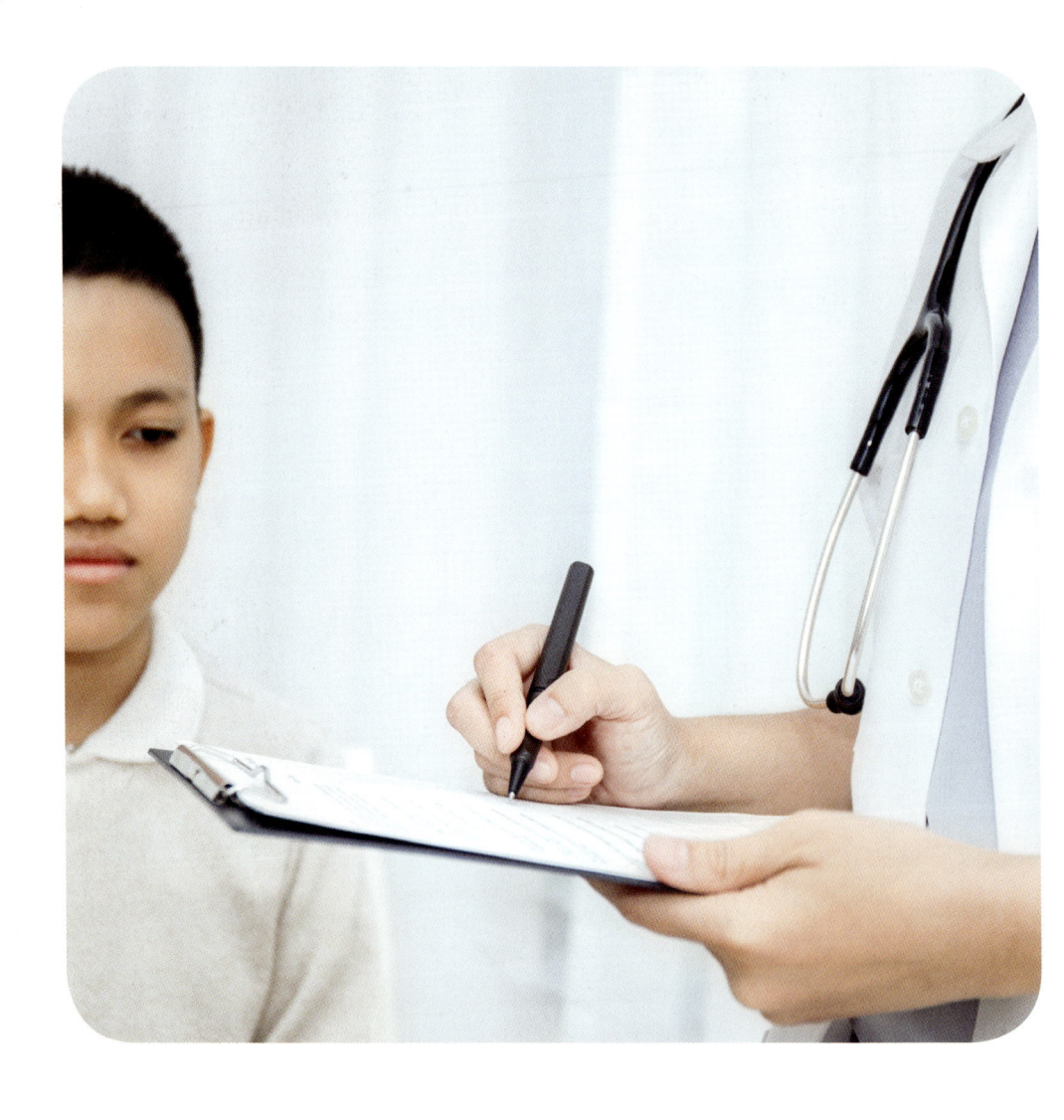

The doctor writes.

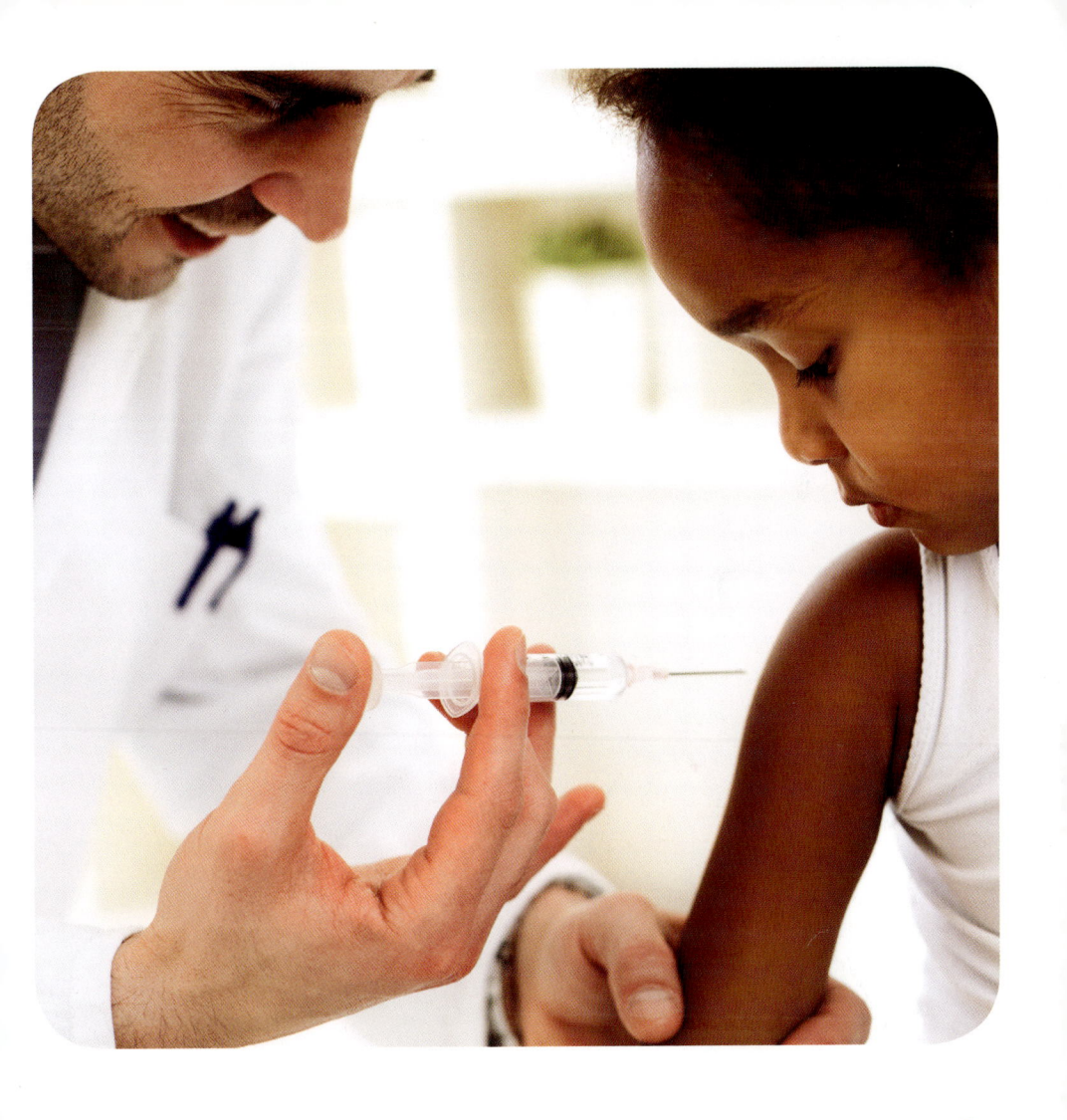

The doctor pokes.

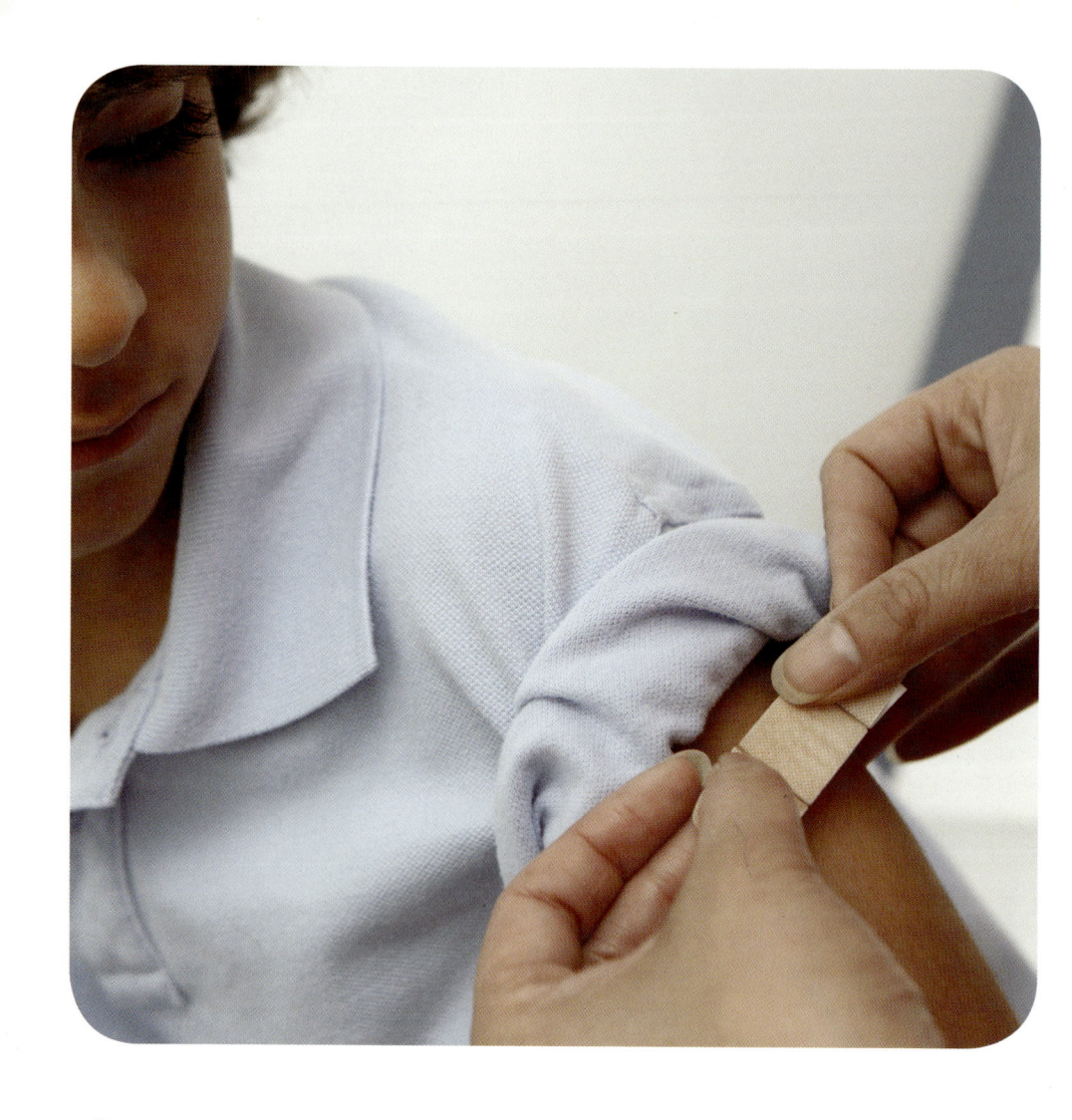

The doctor fixes.

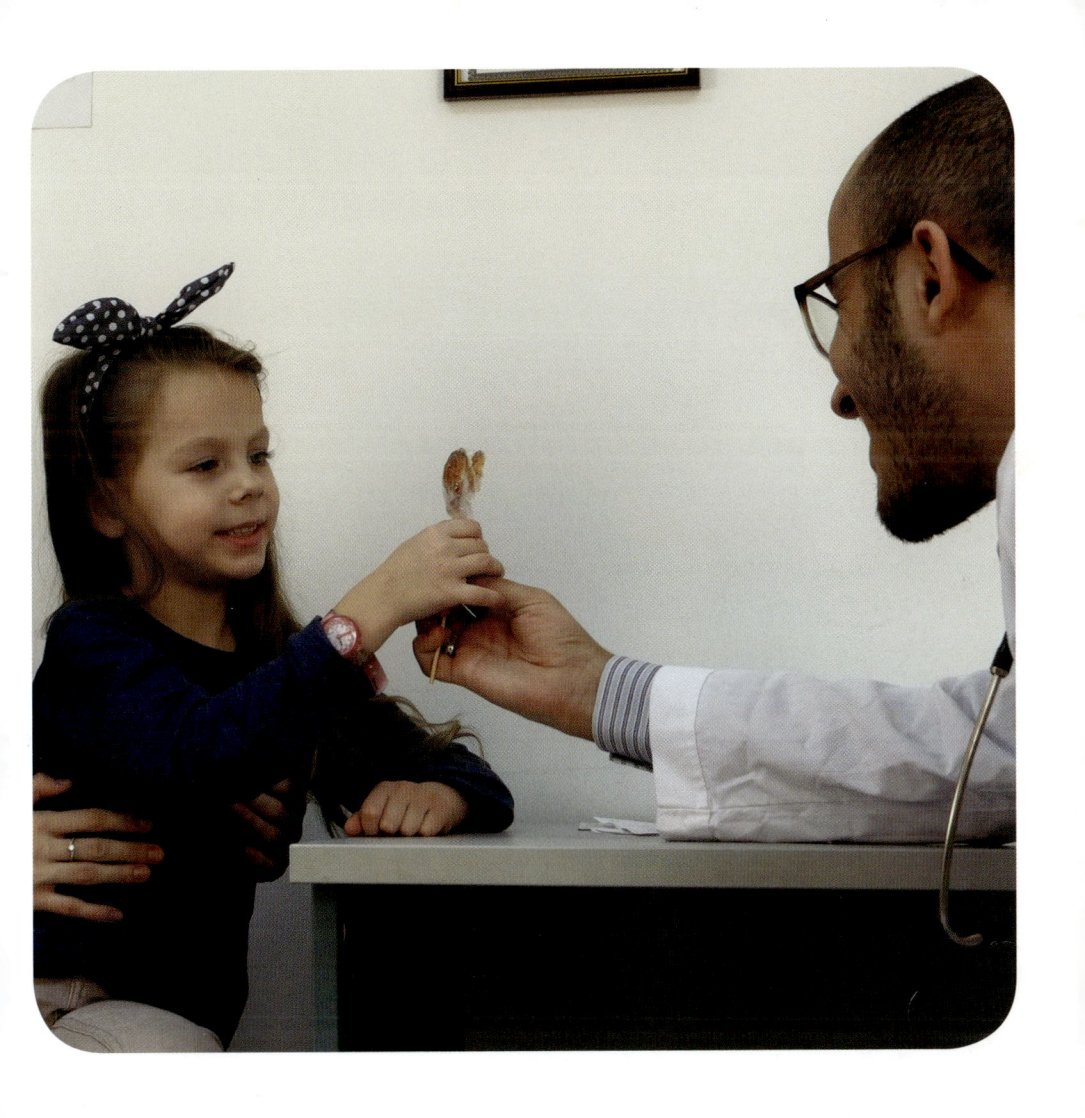

The doctor gives.

# Word List

| | | |
|---|---|---|
| doctor | listens | pokes |
| smiles | squeezes | fixes |
| washes | looks | gives |
| weighs | taps | |
| measures | writes | |

## 36 Words

The doctor smiles.
The doctor washes.
The doctor weighs.
The doctor measures.
The doctor listens.
The doctor squeezes.
The doctor looks.
The doctor taps.
The doctor writes.
The doctor pokes.
The doctor fixes.
The doctor gives.

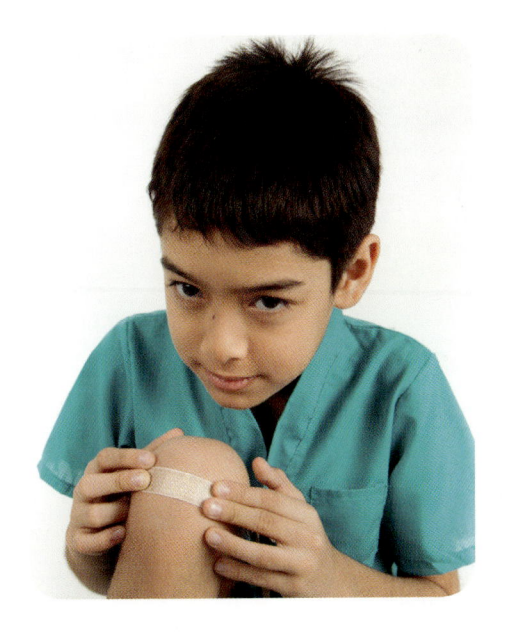

Published in the United States of America by Cherry Lake Publishing
Ann Arbor, Michigan
www.cherrylakepublishing.com

Photo Credits: ©didesign021/shutterstock.com, front cover; ©New Africa/shutterstock.com, 1; ©Photographee.eu/Shutterstock.com, 2; ©YAKOBCHUK VIACHESLAV/Shutterstock.com, 3; ©Rocketclips, Inc. /Shutterstock.com, 4; ©sirtravelalot/Shutterstock.com, 5, 12; ©BlurryMe/Shutterstock.com, 6; ©JPC-PROD/Shutterstock.com, 7; ©Andrey_Popov/Shutterstock.com, 8, 9; ©paulaphoto/Shutterstock.com, 10; ©didesign021/Shutterstock.com, 11; ©Fancy Studio/Shutterstock.com, 13; ©Littlekidmoment/Shutterstock.com, 15, back cover

Copyright © 2020 by Cherry Lake Publishing

All rights reserved. No part of this book may be reproduced or utilized
in any form or by any means without written permission from the publisher.

Cherry Blossom Press is an imprint of Cherry Lake Publishing.

Library of Congress Cataloging-in-Publication Data

Names: Sarantou, Katlin, author.
Title: Visiting the doctor / written by Katlin Sarantou.
Description: Ann Arbor, Michigan : Cherry Lake Publishing, 2020. | Series: Healthy living | Audience: Grades K-1. | Summary: "Learn what the doctor does during a visit to make sure you stay healthy. The book utilizes social emotional based text to get children comfortable with reading, and uses the Whole Language approach to literacy, a combination of sight words and repetition builds recognition and confidence. Bold, colorful photographs correlate directly to text to help guide readers through the book"– Provided by publisher.
Identifiers: LCCN 2019034129 (print) | LCCN 2019034130 (ebook) | ISBN 9781534160958 (paperback) | ISBN 9781534159808 (pdf) | ISBN 9781534162105 (ebook)
Subjects: LCSH: Children–Preparation for medical care–Juvenile literature. | Physicians–Juvenile literature. | Medical care–Juvenile literature. | Readers (Elementary)
Classification: LCC R690 .S27 2020  (print) | LCC R690 (ebook) | DDC 610.69–dc23
LC record available at https://lccn.loc.gov/2019034129
LC ebook record available at https://lccn.loc.gov/2019034130

Printed in the United States of America
Corporate Graphics

CHERRY BLOSSOM PRESS